CW00548097

Bariatric

Cookbook

The bariatric recipe book to enjoy your favorite foods after surgery to lose weight, for a healthy life before and after surgery

The information in the following pages is broadly considered a truthful and accurate account of facts and as such, any inattention, use, or misuse of the information in question by the reader will render any resulting actions solely under their purview. There are no scenarios in which the publisher or the original author of this work can be in any fashion deemed liable for any hardship or damages that may befall them after undertaking information described herein.

Additionally, the information in the following pages is intended only for informational purposes and should thus be thought of as universal. As befitting its nature, it is presented without assurance regarding its prolonged validity or interim quality. Trademarks that are mentioned are done without written consent and can in no way be considered an endorsement from the trademark holder.

CONTENTS

INTRODUCTION

Obesity is characterized as having a weight list (BMI) of at least 30. BMI is a proportion of your weight in connection to your tallness. Class 1 obesity implies a BMI of 30 to 35, Class 2 obesity is a BMI of 35 to 40, and Class 3 obesity is a BMI of at least 40. Classes 2 and 3, otherwise called extreme obesity, are often difficult to treat with diet and exercise alone.

What is bariatric surgery?

Bariatric surgery is an activity that causes you get more fit by making changes to your stomach related framework. A few sorts of bariatric medical procedures make your stomach littler, enabling you to eat and drink less at once and making you feel full sooner. Other bariatric medical procedures likewise change your small digestive system—the piece of your body that assimilates calories and supplements from nourishments and refreshments.

-Bariatric surgery might be an alternative if you have extreme obesity and have not had the option to get more fit or prevent from recovering any weight you lost utilizing different techniques, for example, lifestyle treatment or drugs. Bariatric surgery likewise might be an alternative if you have genuine health issues, for example, type 2 diabetes or rest apnea, identified with obesity. Bariatric surgery can improve a large number of the ailments connected to obesity, particularly type 2 diabetes.

Does bariatric surgery consistently work?

Studies show that numerous individuals who have bariatric surgery lose around 15 to 30 percent of their beginning load by and large, contingent upon the kind of surgery they have. In any case, no strategy, including surgery, makes certain to deliver and keep up weight reduction. A few people who have bariatric surgery may not lose as much as they trusted. After some time, a few people recover a segment of the weight they lost. The measure of weight individuals recapture may shift. Components that influence weight recapture may incorporate an individual's degree of obesity and the sort of surgery the person had.

Bariatric surgery doesn't supplant healthy propensities, however may make it simpler for you to devour less calories and be all the more physically dynamic. Picking healthy nourishments and drinks when the surgery may assist you with losing more weight and keep it off long haul. Normal physical action after surgery additionally helps keep the weight off. To improve your health, you should focus on a lifetime of healthy lifestyle propensities and following the exhortation of your health care suppliers. This book will provide you with the types of food you can eat before and after the surgery.

WHAT YOU SHOULD KNOW BEFORE UNDERGOING BARIATRIC SURGERY

Before you can choose whether this is a decent decision for you, you have to know the realities. In spite of the fact that bariatric surgery is sheltered and by and large effective in accomplishing weight reduction, to be a decent up-and-comer, you should be set up to arrangement with both physical and intense subject matters.

Seven years back, I had a gastric detour and went from being scarcely ready to capacity to carrying on with a magnificent life as an authentic and beneficial individual. (I recount to my story in more profundity at Medium and in my book Recovering My Life: A Personal Bariatric Story.)

All things considered, I talk as a clinician (I am an authorized Marriage and Family Therapist) and as somebody who has experienced weight reduction surgery and the difficult procedure of recuperation. I am not a nutritionist or therapeutic professional.

In any case, my experience and research have instructed me that fruitful bariatric surgery requires arrangement, long haul recuperation, and lifelong changes in your associations with your body, nourishment, and the individuals in your life.

What is bariatric surgery?

Bariatric surgery is definitely not a restorative strategy. We may would like to look better in the wake of getting in shape, yet the best purposes behind experiencing this significant surgery are to expand and improve our lives.

The most well-known strategies are lap band, with a triumph pace of 47%; gastric sleeve, with a triumph pace of 80%; and gastric detour, which has a 85% achievement rate. These systems bolster weight reduction while requiring lifestyle changes.

There's a typical misinterpretation that most patients who have bariatric (weight reduction) surgery recover their weight. Actually, most bariatric surgery patients keep up fruitful weight reduction long haul.

Patients who experience bariatric surgery and pursue all treatment rules can hope to shed pounds and improve the nature of their lives. Over 85% of patients lose and keep up half of their underlying weight reduction.

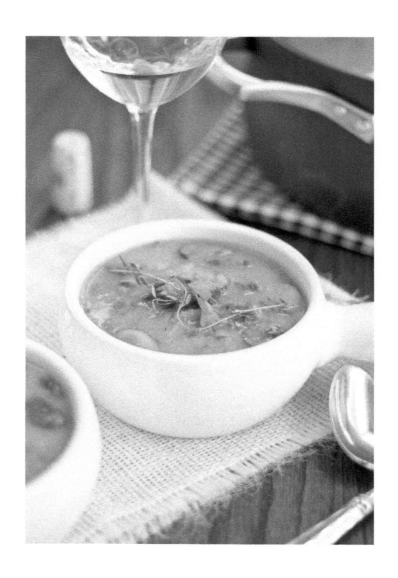

Physical and intense subject matters

If you're considering bariatric surgery, it's critical to get all the data you need—including the physical and enthusiastic high points and low points.

Despite the fact that bariatric surgery is sheltered and less life-compromising than obesity, it is significant surgery. You should manage physical agony, medicine, potential inconveniences, and all the not out of the ordinary issues related with surgery. More, you will confront dietary limitations, some of which are progressing, as not drinking with dinners.

Maybe the more noteworthy test is managing the psychological and intense subject matters. For a considerable length of time, you have utilized nourishment as a methods for adapting.

Changing that confused relationship goes a long ways past returning to "typical" after surgery. The new ordinary will be a novel way to deal with and comprehension of nourishment, your body, and others.

The test of planning for surgery

Convincing and supporting

You should be certain beyond a shadow of a doubt this is the best way for you because you'll need to persuade others: your family, your primary care physicians, and your protection transporter.

To be considered for the surgery, your primary care physician must prescribe it. Then, you should give at any rate a half year of records demonstrating your weight and your endeavors to lose the weight. When you have the specialists ready, your medicinal protection supplier must approve installment.

Upholding for yourself implies teaching yourself, arranging, and figuring out how to support yourself.

Arranging and building support

When you've been affirmed, you have to assemble an emotionally supportive network. One of the most significant choices you'll make is picking your group. The relatives, companions, associates, and experts in your group must regard and bolster your choice.

You'll have to make arrangements for an all-encompassing recuperation. Past help with childcare, family errands, and transportation during and after hospitalization, you will require help acclimating to the adjustments in your life and the feelings that go with those changes.

Your specialist is probably going to expect you to pursue a weight reduction routine for around a half year before surgery to guarantee you are submitted and as healthy as conceivable before surgery.

You'll have to manage fears and dissatisfactions. Backing from a specialist or care group and family is as significant now as it will be later.

The test of recuperation

Recuperation from the surgery itself is only the start.

Physical recuperation

Your primary care physicians will prompt you about the physical difficulties that may pursue bariatric surgery: obstruction, dumping disorder (queasiness, spewing, and shortcoming brought about by eating high sugar dinners, soft drinks, and organic product juices), conceivable disease of the injury, and potential holes in the new associations.

Physical changes may incorporate body hurts or weariness (nutrient or mineral insufficiency might be the reason). You may feel cold. Dry or drooping skin, male pattern baldness or diminishing, and the powerlessness to process certain nutrients (B12 and D) and minerals (iron, folate, calcium) may cause issues.

Drugs

Dealing with your agony prescription is another test. The beginning period of recuperation can last from one to about a month and a half. You should decrease from solution torment drugs. Try not to go without any weaning period!

Pursue your primary care physician's recommendation taking drugs. Halting without therapeutic endorsement can cause genuine intricacies, even hospitalization.

Know that bariatric patients ought not take NSAIDs (nonsteroidal mitigating drugs) like ibuprofen. NSAIDs are undependable for individuals who have experienced bariatric surgery. Indeed, even one use can cause "minimal ulcers", that is, wounds or gaps in the stomach pocket. If it is important to take a NSAID, take it with a proton siphon inhibitor (PPI) medicine, for example, Prilosec or Nexium.

Passionate symptoms

Restorative guidance may not give you the data you need about the enthusiastic reactions of your surgery. You may lose your hunger, or you may feel hungry. You'll be on a fluid eating routine from the start, and that can be distressing.

You may encounter "nourishment sadness". Nourishment has a unique importance for individuals who experience the ill effects of sullen obesity, and "grieving for lost nourishments is a characteristic advance in the re-birth process after weight reduction surgery."

Intense subject matters such as self-uncertainty and emotional episodes may emerge. Weight reduction will be sensational from the start, yet there might be misfortunes—arriving at a level or recapturing some weight.

It might require some investment to become accustomed to your new body. Keep your desires practical. Concentrate on the improvement in your health.

Request help. Set aside effort for self-care. Keep companions who bolster you close. Maintain a strategic distance from the ones who don't. Utilize your emotionally supportive network.

Different dangers

Liquor use

A few patients who have experienced weight reduction surgery battle with liquor and substance misuse. One clarification is "fixation swapping". No longer ready to utilize nourishment as a compulsion, the patient might be attracted to liquor or different substances as substitutes.

Likewise, weight reduction surgery is known to change liquor affectability because the liquor experiences the stomach and into the small digestive tract all the more rapidly. You feel even modest quantities all the more quickly.

Dietary problems

Amusingly, you might be in danger of building up a dietary problem after bariatric surgery. Experiencing difficulty eating because you don't have a craving may prompt "the sort of scattered eating that can transform into bulimia or anorexia."

After surgery, eating too rapidly or not biting altogether can cause spewing. Another unhealthy propensity is biting and letting out nourishment, which can prompt a dietary problem.

Adapting new dietary patterns

Eating out might be a test after bariatric surgery. Keep away from fatty beverages, similar to lattes and soft drinks. Select suppers with an equalization of protein, fiber, and healthy fats. Try not to be reluctant to make your own dish, request a half segment, or take remains.

New dietary patterns to get:

Bite each nibble altogether

Eat gradually

Eat six little suppers rather than three major ones

Quit eating when you feel full

Drink heaps of water (8 cups for each day)

Be set up for change

Bariatric surgery, in any event, when fruitful, orders changes in numerous everyday issues. A considerable lot of these, similar to better health, more vitality, and better confidence, are sure. Be that as it may, despite the fact that your body might be in better health, enthusiastic difficulties may remain.

Missing nourishment and the customs that encompass it, missing old propensities, the pressure of the surgery, and postoperative difficulties may trigger melancholy in certain patients.

Uneasiness after surgery isn't unprecedented.

Patients may end up concentrating on one body part or encountering Body Dysmorphic Disorder (fixating on appearance).

Health issues like recovering weight, the weight reduction level, and complexities from the surgery may emerge.

Hypoglycemia (low glucose), wholesome insufficiencies, and lack of hydration may cause awkward indications and require treatment or changes in diet.

It's dependent upon you to deal with the physical and passionate difficulties. With the assistance of your medicinal group and your care group, you can face these hardships and carry on with the magnificent, gainful life you are intended to live.

Continuous recuperation

Fruitful bariatric surgery implies rolling out lifelong improvements to your lifestyle. Taking on the physical and passionate work to roll out these improvements requires absolute duty to your health. Is it true that you are prepared to address these difficulties? Then you're prepared for bariatric surgery.

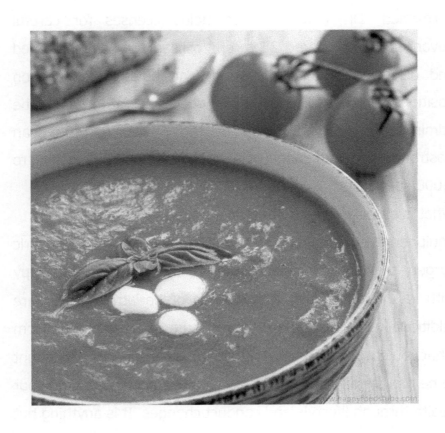

Famous bariatric specialist, researcher, educator and scientist Aurora Pryor, MD, is forming the fate of endoscopic and bariatric surgery — directly here on Long Island. During the most recent 16 years, she has managed in excess of 3,000 careful cases, including 1,000 bariatric techniques she performed. Dr. Pryor likewise holds licenses for careful advances, has prepared 25 careful colleagues, has distributed and displayed around the world, and holds administration positions with conspicuous expert social orders including the administering leading group of the Society of American Gastrointestinal and Endoscopic Surgeons (SAGES), speaking to 6,000 specialists.

What is associated with bariatric surgery?

Equipped to patients who are significantly overweight, bariatric surgery makes the stomach littler so the patient feels happy with less nourishment. A few kinds of bariatric surgery are additionally malabsorptive, so you take in less calories from what you eat. To work most adequately, bariatric surgery ought to be a piece of a continuous adventure toward changing your health through lifestyle and conduct changes. It is anything but a programmed fix.

What is uncommon about Stony Brook's methodology?

We have an uncommon interdisciplinary group of experts who work next to each other with you at all times, sympathetic specialists who truly have any kind of effect. In view of your needs and objectives, your treatment technique may incorporate surgery, restorative administration, diet and exercise, conduct modification and mental guiding. Gathering support incorporates a presurgery medicinally regulated get-healthy plan, just as month to month bolster bunch gatherings after surgery. We keep on meeting with you routinely during the principal year after your surgery, then every year or varying for the remainder of your life. Patients at Stony Brook additionally approach the wide scope of ability, administrations, innovation and offices accessible at Long Island's just scholastic therapeutic focus — which incorporates Suffolk County's just tertiary consideration emergency clinic and Level 1 Trauma Center.

What sorts of bariatric methods are advertised?

We offer the present generally progressed, compelling systems. Most by far are performed laparoscopically, which implies negligible scarring and quicker recuperation.

Customizable Gastric Banding. A silicone band with an infusion port is carefully embedded to make a little pocket of stomach over the band. The band can be balanced during postsurgical office visits utilizing a needle to infuse saline arrangement into the band through the port. The littler stomach makes patients feel full sooner and eat less nourishment.

Banding with Plication. Like movable gastric banding, this methodology diminishes stomach limit without requiring resectioning. It is another and investigational variety that includes collapsing the stomach under the band to decrease it to a sleeve-like pocket.

Sleeve Gastrectomy. The specialist makes a little, sleeve-molded stomach about the size of a banana. It saves the elements of the stomach while seriously diminishing its volume. It might be an independent system or the antecedent to gastric detour in a two-section treatment for patients with a weight record (BMI) of 60 or higher.

Roux-en-Y Gastric Bypass. This method diminishes stomach size while diverting nourishment to sidestep a bit of the small digestive tract, which assimilates calories and supplements. The specialist makes an egg-sized stomach pocket utilizing around five percent of the stomach and afterward connects a Y-molded area of the small digestive system straightforwardly to the pocket.

If you're thinking about weight reduction surgery, there's a decent possibility you're getting a lot of pre-and post-operation direction from a specialist you trust. Yet, that is not generally the situation, and for some individuals who have this sort of method, life after surgery can be brimming with shocks — the great, the terrible, and even the out and out humiliating. If you're considering experiencing bariatric surgery, here are a couple of things you should realize that the specialist may neglect to make reference to.

1. You may get discouraged post-surgery.

There's a demonstrated connection among obesity and despondency, and keeping in mind that most of patients who experience bariatric surgery do encounter a general improvement in their prosperity after surgery, sentiments of wretchedness can compound for a few. Specialists from Yale University distributed an investigation in the Obesity Journal in which 13 percent of patients considered announced an expansion in Beck Depression Inventory – a numerical rating that estimates dietary problem conduct, confidence, and social working – six to a year after gastric detour surgery, a time period that the creators close is a significant period to survey for wretchedness and related manifestations.

2. Abundance skin can be an issue — and restorative surgery is expensive.

In spite of the fact that the post-surgery weight reduction might be continuous enough that your body and skin can alter gradually, numerous individuals are left with such an overabundance, that it requires restorative surgery to fix. Also, except if it's considered restoratively fundamental, (for example, an overflow of saggy skin causing a rash or contamination), your insurance agency won't pay. As per the American Society of Plastic Surgeons, in 2013 part specialists performed about 42,000 body molding tasks — reshaping of bosoms, arms, thighs, and stomachs — for patients who lost considerable measures of weight. Body shaping tasks can cost somewhere in the range of $4,000 to a whole lot higher.

3. You're going to crap more — significantly more.

Around 85 percent of patients who experience Roux-en-Y Gastric Bypass (RNYGB) surgery will encounter outrageous episodes of looseness of the bowels known as dumping disorder sooner or later post-surgery, as indicated by The American Society for Metabolic and Bariatric Surgery (ASMBS). It's normally the aftereffect of poor nourishment decisions (counting refined sugars, seared nourishments, and a few fats or dairy), and can have gentle to-serious side effects that additionally incorporate perspiring, flushing, discombobulation, want to rests, queasiness, squeezing, and dynamic discernible insides sounds. Sound like a bad dream? Tragically, that is not every: Loose stool, blockage, and humiliating gas (or as specialists allude to it, malodorus flatus) are other basic gut related objections after surgery.

4. It could help your hazard for liquor use or misuse.

One examination distributed in JAMA analyzed individuals who had gastric detour surgery at one, three, six, and two years after surgery and found that patients' hazard for expanded liquor use after the method was significantly higher. This might be because patients have higher pinnacle liquor levels, and arrive at those levels all the more rapidly, after bariatric surgery, albeit different speculations do exist to clarify the association.

5. Regardless you'll require that exercise center participation.

Numerous specialists will guide patients on a legitimate post-surgery diet to help advance weight reduction accomplishment after surgery, yet that is not by any means the only lifestyle change patients need to make. The Obesity Action Coalition suggests that once a patient is cleared by their primary care physician to bring physical movement into an everyday schedule, progressively working as long as an hour of activity six days out of each week is perfect for advancing post-surgery weight reduction achievement. As it were, don't believe you're getting off simple; this surgery is anything but a handy solution.

6. You'll need to bid farewell to pop.

The truth is out: Carbonated drinks are a major no-no because they bring air into your gut, making gas that can put pressure on your stomach and cause it to grow superfluously, along these lines fixing the surgery results. Rather than pop, drink parts and loads of water, as drying out is the most widely recognized purpose behind a patient's readmission to the emergency clinic, as indicated by the ASMBS.

7. It could put a strain on your marriage.

Exceptional physical changes can prompt an assortment of enthusiastic changes that can influence you as well as your connections too. At any rate one examination has discovered an uptick in separate from rates among couples with a bariatric surgery accomplice, particularly in the primary year after surgery. So notwithstanding extraordinary post-usable restorative consideration, you additionally may need to consider looking for passionate direction for you and your life partner — either by means of advising with a specialist or by joining a care group, which can help limit the negative consequences for your connections.

8. You could be a possibility for new yearning controlling gadget that can treat obesity.

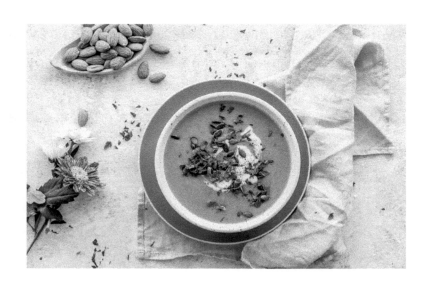

The FDA simply affirmed a first-of-its-sort pacemaker-like weight reduction gadget called the Maestro Rechargeable System, which smothers craving by sending electronic heartbeats to the nerve of the body that conveys appetite to the mind. Despite the fact that less intrusive than bariatric surgery, the gadget requires 60 minutes in length outpatient surgery to embed the gadget in the patient's guts. Since it's not yet broadly accessible, and weight reduction results aren't so amazing as bariatric surgery, it may not swap your requirement for bariatric surgery; still, it could be a decent choice for seriously stout patients who need assistance getting to a weight where they can securely experience bariatric surgery, or for the individuals who need assistance with post-surgery weight control, so it merits talking about with your primary care physician.

9. The dangers of surgery are low contrasted and doing nothing by any means.

In spite of the fact that weight reduction surgery has gained notoriety for being hazardous, the methods have improved throughout the years and are much more secure now; the ASMBS reports that the odds of having a significant confusion are just about 4.3 percent. The dangers of remaining fat — coronary illness, diabetes, stroke, and even passing — are unquestionably progressively hazardous.

10. A great many people say they'd do it again instantly.

Despite the fact that achievement is a long haul venture for patients who experience this genuine system, a great many people say that if they could return in time, they'd decide to have the surgery once more. Numerous individuals report that after the surgery and resulting weight reduction they feel much improved, are increasingly dynamic, and take less prescriptions to treat the intricacies of obesity — all of which can significantly improve an individual's personal satisfaction.

The Bariatric Diet is a Good Eating Plan for Everyone

If you have had gastric detour surgery, you have likely been advised to adhere to a healthy eating regimen so as to hold your weight down as long as possible. A great eating plan post-surgery is known as the bariatric diet. This eating routine, in any case, isn't only for individuals who have experienced bariatric surgeries. It's a decent nourishing arrangement for everybody to pursue.

What Is The Bariatric Diet?

After bariatric surgery, your Atlanta specialist will expect you to hold fast to settling on great nourishment decisions by adhering to an eating regimen that layouts various different stages. The main period of the bariatric diet comprises of clear fluids to keep you hydrated following surgery. This eating regimen can incorporate light, weakened organic product juices, clear juices, water and different nourishments, for example, gelatin or ice pops. The following stage might be a pureed eating regimen enhanced with protein shakes. Following half a month, you would proceed onward to a delicate eating regimen for a few months. This versatile eating regimen will join high protein nourishments and up to 64 ounces of liquids for every day.

At last, the adjustment period of the bariatric diet comprises of eating three nutritious suppers daily and drinking zero-calorie liquids between dinners. This lifelong eating regimen is based after eating lean meats for protein, low-fat dairy things, low-fat grains, and a lot of leafy foods. This is a magnificent lifelong eating regimen for any individual who wishes to stay healthy and thin.

Why the Bariatric Diet Is a Healthy Way of Eating

Patients in the Atlanta region who have experienced bariatric surgery comprehend the significance of keeping up their weight and controlling segment sizes. This specific eating regimen, in its standardization stage, shows you what and how to eat notwithstanding helping you keep your weight stable.

The bariatric diet is a high-protein, low-starch, low-sugar wholesome arrangement. You center around eating healthy nourishments and proteins first, with negligible nibbling between dinners. Rather, drinking water and other without calorie fluids are empowered.

There is a sure method for eating your suppers on this eating routine. When devouring your supper, for example, decide to eat the lean protein on your plate first. This might be a bit of lean meat with any fat expelled, chicken with no skin, eggs, or fish. Next, eat the vegetables or natural product, lastly proceed onward to expending whatever starch or grain (sugar) is on your plate. Downplay sugars and eat three suppers every day, with a couple of little snacks in the middle of dinners if you need them. These bites ought to be low in carbs, high in protein, low in sugar.

This nourishment plan will keep you healthy while enabling you to keep up your present weight. Make sure to eat gradually and bite each chomp totally. Making sure to quit eating once you feel full is significant. Inquire as to whether you're as yet eager. If you're not, then quit eating. Keeping up your liquid admission between suppers is additionally significant for keeping up supplements in travel to your organs and keeping you hydrated. Take a multi-nutrient day by day.

Gastric detour diet: What to eat after the surgery

Thinking about what your eating regimen will resemble after your surgery? Realize which nourishments will assist you with recuperating and get in shape securely.

A gastric detour diet helps individuals who are recouping from sleeve gastrectomy and from gastric detour surgery — otherwise called Roux-en-Y gastric detour — to recuperate and to change their dietary patterns.

Your primary care physician or an enlisted dietitian will converse with you about the eating routine you'll have to trail surgery, clarifying what sorts of nourishment and the amount you can eat at every dinner. Firmly following your gastric detour diet can assist you with getting more fit securely.

Reason

The gastric detour diet is intended to:

Enable your stomach to mend without being extended by the nourishment you eat

Get you used to eating the littler measures of nourishment that your littler stomach can easily and securely digest

Assist you with getting in shape and abstain from putting on weight

Maintain a strategic distance from symptoms and intricacies from the surgery

Diet subtleties

Diet proposals after gastric detour surgery change contingent upon your individual circumstance.

A gastric detour diet commonly pursues an organized way to deal with assistance you move over into eating strong nourishments. How rapidly you move starting with one stage then onto the next relies upon how quick your body recuperates and acclimates to the adjustment in eating designs. You can ordinarily begin eating ordinary nourishments around a quarter of a year after surgery.

At each phase of the gastric detour diet, you should be mindful so as to:

Drink 64 ounces of liquid daily, to maintain a strategic distance from lack of hydration.

Taste fluids between suppers, not with dinners. Hold up around 30 minutes after a dinner to drink anything and abstain from drinking 30 minutes before a supper.

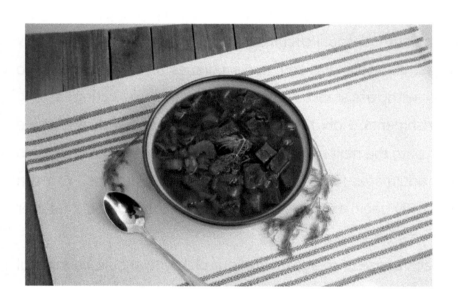

Eat and drink gradually, to abstain from dumping disorder —
which happens when nourishments and fluids enter your small
digestive system quickly and in bigger sums than typical,
causing sickness, spewing, wooziness, perspiring and loose
bowels.

Eat lean, protein-rich nourishments day by day.

Pick nourishments and beverages that are low in fats and sugar.

Dodge liquor.

Point of confinement caffeine, which can cause drying out.

Take nutrient and mineral enhancements day by day as
coordinated by your health supplier.

Bite nourishments altogether to a pureed consistency before
gulping, when you progress past fluids as it were.

Fluids

For the primary day or so after surgery, you'll just be permitted
to drink clear fluids. When you're taking care of clear fluids, you
can begin having different fluids, for example,

Stock

Unsweetened juice

Decaffeinated tea or espresso

Milk (skim or 1 percent)

Without sugar gelatin or popsicles

Pureed nourishments

After about seven days of enduring fluids, you can start to eat stressed and pureed (squashed up) nourishments. The nourishments ought to have the consistency of a smooth glue or a thick fluid, with no strong bits of nourishment in the blend. You can eat three to six little dinners daily. Every dinner should comprise of 4 to 6 tablespoons of nourishment. Eat gradually — around 30 minutes for every feast.

Pick nourishments that will puree well, for example,

Lean ground meat, poultry or fish

Curds

Delicate fried eggs

Cooked grain

Delicate leafy foods vegetables

Stressed cream soups

Mix strong nourishments with a fluid, for example,

Water

Skim milk

Juice with no sugar included

Juices

Delicate nourishments

Following half a month of pureed nourishments, and with your primary care physician's OK, you can add delicate nourishments to your eating routine. They ought to be little, delicate and effectively bit bits of nourishment.

You can eat three to five little dinners daily. Every dinner should comprise of 33% to one-half cup of nourishment. Bite each chomp until the nourishment is pureed consistency before gulping.

Delicate nourishments include:

Ground lean meat or poultry

Chipped fish

Eggs

Curds

Cooked or dried oat

Rice

Canned or delicate crisp natural product, without seeds or skin

Cooked vegetables, without skin

Strong nourishments

After around about two months on the gastric detour diet, you can step by step come back to eating firmer nourishments. Start with eating three dinners per day, with every feast comprising of 1 to 1-1/2 cups of nourishment. It's imperative to quit eating before you feel totally full.

Contingent upon how you endure strong nourishment, you might have the option to change the quantity of dinners and measure of nourishment at every supper. Converse with your dietitian about what's best for you.

Attempt new nourishments each in turn. Certain nourishments may cause agony, queasiness or regurgitating after gastric detour surgery.

Nourishments that can cause issues at this stage include:

Breads

Carbonated beverages

Crude vegetables

Cooked sinewy vegetables, for example, celery, broccoli, corn or cabbage

Intense meats or meats with cartilage

Red meat

Singed nourishments

Exceptionally prepared or fiery nourishments

Nuts and seeds

Popcorn

After some time, you may have the option to attempt a portion of these nourishments once more, with the direction of your primary care physician.

Another healthy eating regimen

Gastric detour surgery lessens the size of your stomach and changes the manner in which nourishment enters your digestive organs. After surgery, it's essential to get sufficient sustenance while keeping your weight reduction objectives on track. Your PCP is probably going to suggest that you:

Eat and drink gradually. To abstain from dumping disorder, take in any event 30 minutes to eat your dinners and 30 to an hour to drink 1 cup of fluid. Hold up 30 minutes prior or after every dinner to drink fluids.

Keep dinners little. Eat a few little suppers daily. You may begin with six little suppers daily, then move to four dinners lastly, when following a customary eating routine, three dinners every day. Every feast ought to incorporate about a half-cup to 1 cup of nourishment.

Drink fluids between suppers. To maintain a strategic distance from lack of hydration, you'll have to drink in any event 8 cups (1.9 liters) of liquids daily. Be that as it may, drinking an excessive amount of fluid at or around supper time can leave you feeling excessively full and keep you from eating enough supplement rich nourishment.

Bite nourishment altogether. The new opening that leads from your stomach into your small digestive system is thin and can be obstructed by bigger parts of nourishment. Blockages keep nourishment from leaving your stomach and can cause regurgitating, sickness and stomach torment. Take little chomps of nourishment and bite them to a pureed consistency before gulping.

Concentrate on high-protein nourishments. Eat these nourishments before you eat different food sources in your supper.

Keep away from nourishments that are high in fat and sugar. These nourishments travel rapidly through your stomach related framework and cause dumping disorder.

Take prescribed nutrient and mineral enhancements. After surgery your body won't have the option to assimilate enough supplements from your nourishment. You'll likely need to take a multivitamin supplement each day for the remainder of your life.

Results

The gastric detour diet can assist you with recouping from surgery and change to a method for eating that is healthy and bolsters your weight reduction objectives. Recollect that if you come back to unhealthy dietary patterns after weight reduction surgery, you may not lose the entirety of your overabundance weight, or you may recover any weight that you do lose.

Risks

The greatest risks of the gastric bypass diet come from not following the diet properly. If you eat too much or eat food that you shouldn't, you could have complications. These include:

Dumping syndrome. If too much food enters your small intestine quickly, you are likely to experience nausea, vomiting, dizziness, sweating and diarrhea. Eating too much or too fast, eating foods high in fat or sugar, and not chewing your food adequately can all cause nausea or vomiting after meals.

Dehydration. Because you're not supposed to drink fluids with your meals, some people become dehydrated. That's why you need to sip 64 ounces (1.9 liters) of water and other fluids throughout the day.

Constipation. A lack of physical activity and of fiber or fluid in your diet can cause constipation.

Blocked opening of your stomach pouch. Food can become lodged at the opening of your stomach pouch, even if you carefully follow the diet. Signs and symptoms of a blocked stomach opening include ongoing nausea, vomiting and abdominal pain. Call your doctor if you have these symptoms for more than two days.

Weight gain or failure to lose weight. If you continue to gain weight or fail to lose weight on the gastric bypass diet, talk to your doctor or dietitian.

THE IMPORTANCE OF
BARIATRIC DIET

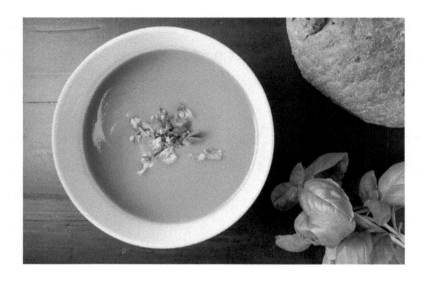

Gastric detour isn't for everybody. You should initially qualify for the surgery and comprehend the dangers and advantages included. The individuals who are qualified are normally in excess of 100 pounds overweight or have a weight list (BMI) more than 40. You may likewise be qualified if your BMI is somewhere in the range of 35 and 40 and your health is in danger because of your weight.

To be a practical up-and-comer, you ought to likewise be prepared to relearn your dietary propensities. New dietary propensities can support the surgery have positive and lifelong impacts.

Prior to your surgery, you have to make arrangements for an extraordinary eating regimen to pursue when the surgery. The presurgery diet is equipped towards lessening the measure of fat in and around your liver. This lessens the danger of confusions during the surgery. After the surgery, your primary care physician with tailor the general eating regimen rules to you. The eating routine comprises of a few week after week stages. It encourages you recoup, address the issues of your now-littler stomach, and addition healthier dietary patterns.

Diet before your surgery

Getting more fit before surgery lessens the measure of fat in and around your liver and belly. This may enable you to have a laparoscopy as opposed to open surgery. Laparoscopic surgery is less intrusive. It requires substantially less recuperation time and is simpler on your body.

Getting thinner preceding surgery keeps you more secure during the methodology, yet it likewise helps train you for another method for eating. It is a lifelong change.

Your definite eating plan and preop weight reduction objective will be dictated by your primary care physician. Your eating plan may start when you are cleared for the system. If adequate weight reduction doesn't happen, the technique might be dropped or deferred. Along these lines, you should begin the eating routine arrangement when you can.

Rules

Rules shift from individual to individual, yet may incorporate the accompanying:

Dispense with or decline soaked fats, including entire milk items, greasy meat, and singed nourishment.

Take out or decline nourishments that are high in starches, for example, sugary pastries, pasta, potatoes, bread, and bread items.

Wipe out high-sugar drinks, for example, juice and soft drinks.

Exercise partition control.

Maintain a strategic distance from voraciously consuming food.

Try not to smoke cigarettes.

Maintain a strategic distance from mixed drinks and recreational medications.

Try not to drink refreshments with your suppers.

Take a day by day multivitamin.

Take protein supplements as protein shakes or powder.

What to eat

The pre-operation diet comprises generally of protein shakes and other high-protein, low-calorie nourishments that are anything but difficult to process. Protein helps reinforce and ensure muscle tissue. This can enable your body to consume fat rather than muscle for fuel. Protein likewise helps keep your body solid, which can accelerate recuperation.

As the date for your surgery approaches, you may need to pursue a for the most part fluid or fluid just diet. In light of your weight and generally health, your primary care physician may enable you to eat a few solids during this time. These might incorporate fish, watered-down hot oat, or delicate bubbled eggs.

Prior to the surgery, ensure you chat with the anesthesiologist for guidelines about what you can or can't have before the surgery. These proposals are evolving. They may need you to drink sugar rich liquids as long as two hours before surgery.

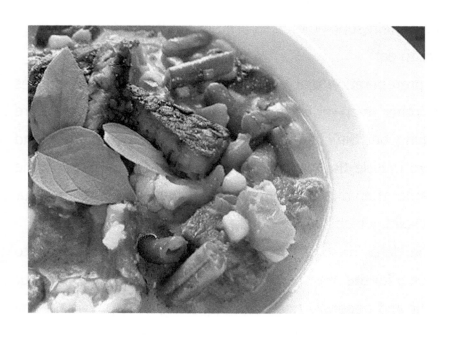

Diet after your surgery

After surgery, the eating routine arrangement experiences a few phases. To what extent each stage endures and what you can eat and drink will be dictated by your primary care physician or dietitian. All stages pressure the significance of bit control. This propensity will assist you with continueing to get in shape and set you up for how you will eat for the remainder of your life.

Stage one: Liquid eating routine

During stage one, your nourishing admission is equipped towards helping your body mend from surgery. Your eating routine can assist you with maintaining a strategic distance from postoperative confusions. For the initial not many days, you are just permitted to drink a couple of ounces of clear fluids one after another. This enables your stomach to mend without being loosened up by nourishment. After clear fluids, you will graduate to extra sorts of fluid. These include:

decaffeinated espresso and tea

skim milk

slender soup and juices

unsweetened juice

sans sugar gelatin

sans sugar popsicles

Stage two: Pureed diet

When your primary care physician chooses you're prepared, you can proceed onward to arrange two. This stage comprises of pureed nourishments that have a thick, pudding-like consistency. Numerous nourishments can be pureed at home with a nourishment processor, blender, or other gadget.

Fiery seasonings may bother the stomach, so stay away from these totally or attempt them each in turn. Maintain a strategic distance from natural products that have bunches of seeds, for example, strawberries or kiwi. You ought to likewise avoid nourishments that are too sinewy to even think about liquefying, for example, broccoli and cauliflower.

V-8 juice and first-organize infant nourishments, which don't contain solids, are likewise helpful choices.

As you begin to incorporate purees into your eating routine, it's significant not to drink liquids while you eat.

Stage three: Soft diet

You will most likely eat only pureed nourishment for a little while. When your primary care physician chooses you're prepared, you can begin fabricating delicate, simple to-bite nourishments into your eating routine. These may include:

delicate bubbled eggs

ground meat

cooked white fish

canned organic products, for example, peaches or pears

It is imperative to eat little chomps. Utilize great segment control and eat a little at once.

Stage four: Stabilization

Stage four of the gastric detour diet incorporates the reintroduction of strong nourishment. It normally starts around two months after surgery. You will in any case need to dice or hack your nourishment into little chomps because your stomach is a lot littler. Enormous bits of nourishment may cause a blockage. A blockage can prompt torment, sickness, and retching.

Present nourishments gradually. That way, you can best figure out which ones your stomach can endure and which ones to stay away from. Dispose of any nourishment that causes stomach distress, spewing, or sickness.

Nourishments to maintain a strategic distance from in arrange four

Certain nourishments ought not be endeavored at this point, for example, food sources that are difficult to process. These include:

sinewy or stringy vegetables, for example, pea pods

popcorn

old fashioned corn

carbonated refreshments, for example, seltzer

intense meat

singed nourishment

crunchy nourishments, for example, pretzels, granola, seeds, and nuts

dried organic product

bread and bread items, for example, biscuits

Around four months after surgery, you might have the option to continue eating typically. Nonetheless, divide control is as yet significant. Ensure your eating routine comprises for the most part of natural products, vegetables, lean protein, and healthy sugars. Dodge unhealthy nourishments that are high in fat, starches, and calories. Eating admirably implies you can appreciate proceeded with health without returning load on.

By and large rules for postop diet

The rules for your postoperative eating routine will likewise serve you all through life. They include:

Eat and drink gradually.

Exercise divide control.

Tune in to your body. If you can't endure a nourishment, for example, something zesty or seared, don't eat it.

Keep away from high-fat and high-sugar nourishments.

Appreciate drinks between suppers, yet not during dinners.

Drink enough every day to maintain a strategic distance from drying out.

Eat just little bits of nourishment at once, and bite each piece completely.

Take the nutrients your PCP suggests.

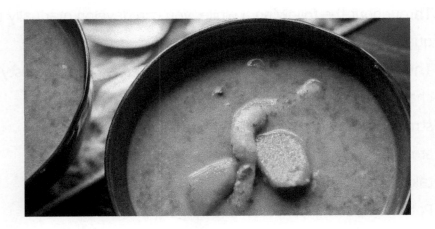

You may feel propelled to start or resume an activity program. Directly after surgery, you have to allow your body to recuperate. Go gradually.

For the principal month, low-sway practices are a decent choice. These incorporate strolling and swimming. You may likewise profit by straightforward yoga stances, extending, and profound breathing activities.

Throughout the following a while, you can develop gradually to quality preparing and cardio exercises.

Think regarding development just as exercise. Basic lifestyle changes can be physical wellness promoters, for example,

strolling as opposed to riding the transport

stopping more remote away from your goal

taking the stairs rather than the lift

Potential inconveniences of the surgery

Following the best possible pre-and post-surgery slims down causes you keep away from inconveniences, for example, lack of hydration, queasiness, and blockage.

Obstacle

Now and again the association between your stomach and digestive organs can get limited. This can happen regardless of whether you are cautious about what you eat. If you have sickness, spewing, or stomach torment for over two days, let your primary care physician know. These are on the whole indications of a check.

Dumping disorder

Bit control and eating and drinking gradually additionally help you keep away from what's called dumping disorder. Dumping disorder happens if nourishments or drinks enter your small digestive tract too rapidly or in too-enormous sums. Eating and drinking simultaneously may likewise cause dumping disorder. This is because it builds consumption volume.

Dumping disorder can occur at any phase of the postop diet. Manifestations include:

perspiring

queasiness

spewing

tipsiness

looseness of the bowels

To help abstain from dumping disorder, a great dependable guideline is to take in any event thirty minutes to eat every feast. Pick low-fat and low-or no-sugar nourishments. Stick around 30 to 45 minutes before drinking any fluids, and consistently taste fluids gradually.

BARIATRIC BREAKFAST RECIPES

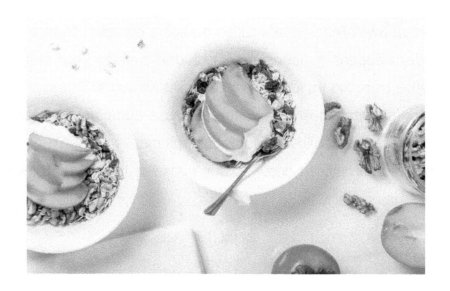

Breakfast is a significant feast. It isn't pretty much significant than lunch or supper, yet breakfast gets investigated more often than some other dinner of the day.

"I don't wake up so as to cook in the first part of the day."

"Espresso is my morning meal."

"I can scarcely get myself and my children out the entryway in the first part of the day on schedule. No way there is the ideal opportunity for breakfast."

It doesn't make a difference what your reason is for avoiding this dinner, chances are I've heard it. What's more, a reason is only that. A reason. In any case, it doesn't change the way that you need great nourishment to improve your center, look after vitality, and control hunger for the duration of the day.

However, since this feast is by all accounts the most difficult for individuals to eat, it merits somewhat more individualized consideration. You will be increasingly disposed to have breakfast if you anticipate incredible plans so we have incorporated a rundown of some extraordinary breakfast thoughts. Every one of these morning meal thoughts are bariatric consistent (some with minor modifications).

BLUEBERRY —ALMOND OVERNIGHT OATS

This no cook formula is too easy to prepare ahead the prior night and impeccable when the climate is hot and you don't want to cook over a hot stove.

I love that you can make a bunch on feast prep Sunday with your preferred flavors.

Blueberries are my child's preferred summer berry. He can eat them by the fistful and hurling a couple into these blueberry medium-term oats consistently carries a major grin to his face.

WHAT DO I NEED TO MAKE OVERNIGHT OATS:

All you have to make medium-term oats are only a couple of basic wash room fixings:

Oats: Overnight oats are ordinarily made with antiquated moved oats and in some cases fast oats. Use gluten free varying.

Chia Seeds: Chia seeds give medium-term oats that thick pudding-like surface and include additional fiber however don't hesitate to forget about them if you aren't a fan.

Milk: Use your preferred dairy or sans dairy milk you like or have close by. We typically prefer to utilize almond however coconut milk, cashew milk all work incredible for a veggie lover alternative.

Yogurt – You can include a blend of milk and yogurt to make your oats extra velvety .

Natural product: Have fun with your fixings. Include organic product that won't get soft legitimately into the artisan container or hurl them on straightforwardly over the oats when you're prepared to eat.

Sugar: Leave out or utilize any sugar you like – nectar, maple syrup, a ready banana, dates or any low-carb fluid sugar like stevia, priest organic product or erythritol will work.

Nut or seed spread: Almond margarine, cashew margarine, pumpkin margarine, sunflower seed spread and additionally nutty spread include that appetizing nutty flavor and a specific smoothness.

INSTRUCTIONS TO MAKE BLUEBERRY OVERNIGHT OATS:

These blueberry medium-term oats are perhaps the most straightforward breakfast that even your children can assist you with amassing the prior night. You can utilize a bricklayer container, resealable compartment or a bowl.

Start by joining rolled or antiquated oats with your preferred milk and/or coconut or Greek yogurt in a 8 oz. artisan container, resealable holder or a bowl. These 7 oz containers are the ones you really find in the photographs and are right now my preferred ones.

Include a couple of blueberries, vanilla and almond spread and blend to consolidate.

Seal up the holder and park it in the cooler medium-term.

The following morning, you can warm the glass container up in the microwave for a blistering breakfast or make the most of your medium-term oats cold directly from the ice chest. You can include more milk and any fun fixings of your decision.

FOR SUNDAY MEAL PREP:

Twofold or triple the bunch and partition into discrete bricklayer containers or resealable compartments.

OTHER FLAVOR OPTIONS FOR OVERNIGHT OATS:

You can include some coconut, lemon, nectar, maple syrup or include a couple of cuts of bananas for additional sweetness and potassium.

Present with strawberries and blackberries for a triple berry treat.

Fixings

½ cup moved oats

½ cup almond milk

2 tablespoon almond spread

½ teaspoon vanilla concentrate

½ teaspoon ground cinnamon

1 cup solidified highbush blueberries, partitioned

1 tablespoon toasted cut almonds

Guidelines

In artisan container join oats, almond milk, almond margarine, vanilla and cinnamon.

Mix in ½ cup blueberries.

Top with remaining ½ cup blueberries and cut almonds.

Spread. Refrigerate 4 hours-medium-term.

Eat up.

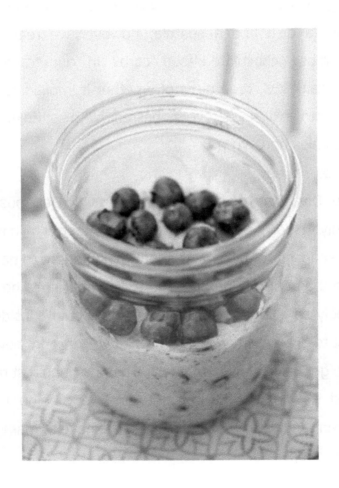

PROTEIN PANCAKES

Flapjacks! Hotcakes! Hotcakes!

With nutty spread and chocolate chips and a smidgen of maple syrup, which is exactly how I gobbled them growing up, post-swimming club practice, once in a while mushed together into a major heap of "mixed flapjacks" because me and my high school squad didn't have a clue what we were in any event, doing with a dish and a spatula, however we realized we required those chocolate-kissed carbs in our frameworks quickly, detail, SOS, regardless of whether it implied squished together into skillet leftovers bested with sprinkles and chocolate chips and syrup.

This is, resurrected.

Grown up. Diva Status. Healthier. Progressively Delicious.

Additionally: I don't generally swim any longer. I'm having a mid-post snapshot of bitterness about that. I ought to get once more into the pool routine once more, isn't that so? The water is genuinely so cold here and there that I would consider not going just to prevent my body from solidifying strong, however, I ought to get back in. Swimming gave me the hungriest hunger ever, and nowadays with my *literal* work being making nourishment and eating? Truly and yes. We have to make these two things cooperate.

Almost certain I once wore a shirt that said swimming is life, the rest is simply subtleties. Anybody? Unexpectedly this is still valid for despite everything me with the exception of it's about nourishment. Nourishment is life and the rest is simply subtleties and PLEASE somebody make that into the up and coming gen of those shirts. I will be at the front of the line when you dispatch.

Companions, may the chances be ever in support of you to have protein flapjacks for breakfast throughout the entire summer. So you can swim or get your mind and body fueled up do whatever else it is that you do.

Like, simply attempt to take a gander at this and disclose to me it doesn't search bravo

Folks. I implied EMOTIONALLY bravo, alright? Relax.

So perhaps I am not saying these are the healthiest hotcakes that at any point lived, yet relying upon how over the edge or not over the edge you go with the garnishes, they could be. We're working with solid potential here.

Tune in to this — these protein flapjacks all alone have no refined sugar because banana has your back. Additionally — no refined grains with an extraordinary s/o to oats on that one. Parcels and parts and heaps of protein — from protein powder if you need (I utilize this collagen protein that a couple of companions prescribed to me, and Bjork utilizes some sort of seasoned whey protein that I turn my nose up to a smidgen, and everybody has their very own inclinations for these things, correct? so I state simply pick on that works for you and continue ahead with your hotcake self) or potentially protein just from the eggs and egg whites. This is an everybody wins club.

Mix that child up and fry on a hot frying pan. Like so

Also, if you halted there, you'd have yourself a pretty epically healthy protein flapjack breakfast. You'd most likely be the sort of purposeful #fitspo individual to top it with organic product, yogurt (weird yet I love it as a healthy garnish because it assists hotcakes with getting that doused syrup-surface without all the sugar), and granola for crunch. GO YOU! We're glad.

Obviously, if you didn't stop there, you would be my protein hotcakes soul sister and you would sit with me and eat the pastry variant of protein flapjacks while rooting for the sisters from situation number one. Is it true that you are getting what I'm putting down? Nutty spread, chocolate chips both IN the flapjacks and on top, and a shower of maple syrup to balance the Breakfast Dessert Masterpiece. There simply is no other path for me.

Protein hotcakes = the new breakfast on the square. also, I am loving this beginner A LOT.

Protein Pancakes! very simple with no refined grains or refined sugar. just oats, banana, and eggs!

Fixings

1 cup oats

1 banana

2 eggs

1/2 cup egg whites

4 teaspoons heating powder

a spot of salt

a spot of cinnamon

1–2 scoops protein powder

2 tablespoons flax feast

Guidelines

Run everything through the blender on medium low speed until very much blended.

Warmth a nonstick iron to medium high warmth. Include hitter in little circles – around 1/4 cup for every flapjack. Sprinkle with blueberries or chocolate chips if you need. When the edges begin to look dry (2-3 minutes), flip and cook one more moment or two on the opposite side.

Top with anything you like! I like syrup and nutty spread and chocolate chips

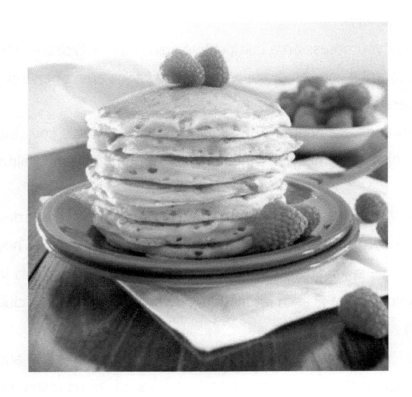

SHAKSHUKA EGG BAKE

The best heated eggs on the planet – Shakshuka! A Middle Eastern and North African dish generally served up for breakfast or lunch, this can be made altogether on the stove or completed in the broiler. In any case, bread for dunking/cleaning isn't discretionary!

I'll give you access on a competitive advantage – typically, the photographs you see of supposed heated eggs aren't generally prepared by any means.

When eggs are heated, the slight film of egg whites covering the yolks gets misty, hazing up the beautiful brilliant yellow yolks.

"This is a calamity!" said some nourishment magazine supervisor, some place. "We can't have foggy yolks! They should be splendid yellow. This must be fixed!" (I hear this in my mind with a French intonation, however I don't have a clue why)

Thus some nourishment beautician abandoned off, and returned with an answer currently embraced by nourishment beauticians all over: sauté the eggs just right then slide them into whatever sauce or vehicle they were as far as anyone knows heated in.

It's constantly evident when this is done because you don't get the untidy seep of whites blended in with the sauce, similar to you find in these photographs.

So truly, I sacrificed incredibly yellow yolks to make this the manner in which the formula is composed. I cheated a piece however I painstakingly cleared off as a significant part of the egg whites from the yolks before preparing them.

I guarantee you I don't do that, in actuality.

Since I've changed the manner in which you'll take a gander at prepared eggs photographs everlastingly, how about we talk about the world's best heated eggs – Shakshuka.

WHAT IS SHAKSHUKA?

It's essentially eggs that are prepared or poached in a fragrant tomato sauce, as a rule with capsicum (ringer peppers), onion and flavors like cumin and paprika, mirroring the Middle Eastern and North African underlying foundations of this dish. It's quite like Huevos Ranchos – the Mexican form of Shakshuka!

In spite of the fact that generally thought of as a morning meal or informal breakfast formula, I'm everlastingly on my "eggs whenever of the day" campaign and I'm staying here at 5.18pm on Wednesday 25 July 2018, thinking about what to have for supper today around evening time and I simply chose to make this (once more).

SPLENDID FOR CAMPING – AND MAKING IN BULK

In spite of the fact that I call Shakshuka a kind of heated eggs, incidentally my preferred method for making it is over open air fire, poaching as opposed to preparing. Probably the closest companion had a remote wild-waterway wedding and the outside cooks they employed made Shakshuka for 80 wedding visitors over open air fire.

It worked splendidly because eggs take negligible minutes to cook, so they made enormous pots of this fragrant tomato sauce then cooked handfuls and many eggs in them. Poach, serve, then rehash in similar pots.

I had every single sincere goal of making a difference. Be that as it may, I had an irritated head that morning... 🍴🌑 Hey! I was a bridesmaid – I needed to do heaps of toasts!

Fixings

2 tbsp olive oil

1 little red onion , stripped, divided and cut

1 garlic clove , minced

1 little red capsicum (ringer pepper) , split lengthways and cut into 0.5cm/1/4" strips

1 tomato , diced

400 g/14 oz can squashed tomatoes

1 tbsp tomato glue

1/2 cup/125 ml chicken or vegetable stock (or water)

1 tsp EACH paprika and cumin

1/4 tsp EACH dark pepper and cayenne pepper (or other hot zest, change in accordance with taste)

1/2 tsp salt

4 eggs (up to 6 eggs alright)

2 tbsp crisp parsley or coriander/cilantro , generally hacked

Pita or dry bread, to serve

Guidelines

Preheat broiler to 180C/350F (if meaning to prepare them).

Warmth oil in a medium size cast iron skillet over medium high warmth. Include garlic and onion, cook for 2 minutes until onion is translucent.

Include capsicum, cook for 1 moment. Include diced tomato, cook for 2 minutes until separated and it turns into somewhat pale (see video).

Include canned tomatoes, tomato glue, juices, paprika, cumin, salt and pepper. Blend to consolidate well.

Lower stove to medium low and stew for 5 minutes until sufficiently thickened to make spaces (don't need dry slop, needs to in any case be saucy).

Make spaces in the blend and cautiously split the eggs in. Leave to cook for 1 moment until edges of whites are set (Note 1).

Move to stove and heat for 7 to 12 minutes until whites are simply set yet yolks are as yet runny (or to your taste). Or then again spread with top and steam on stove for 3 minutes (runny yolks), or simply stew them without a cover.

Expel from broiler/stove and serve promptly, dissipated with the coriander or parsley. Present with dried up bread, or pita bread.

Formula Notes:

1. Preparing eggs splendidly so you get runny yolks however the whites are simply set instead of jam like (ie still a little piece crude) is in reality a touch of a craftsmanship. My method for getting around this is to leave the eggs to cook in the blend for 1 moment before moving to the broiler. This gives the whites somewhat of a head start without influencing the yolks.

2. Varieties - this formula fits a large number of varieties. Take a stab at subbing the capsicum with different vegetables, for example, zucchini (courgettes), eggplants (aubergines), or even carrots or fennel. For a prepared beans-ish turn (that is breakfast heated beans, as Aussies and Poms know them, not American prepared beans), have a go at including white beans. Take a stab at including olives, or other appetizer ey things (artichokes, sun dried tomatoes). For a Mexican turn, use corn and dark beans!

3. This formula as composed makes 2 liberal servings (2 eggs for each individual) (this is the thing that the nourishment reflects). Be that as it may, there's sufficient sauce here for 3 servings if you can crush 6 eggs in. I selected to simply utilize 4 here so you can really observe the sauce in the photographs and video.

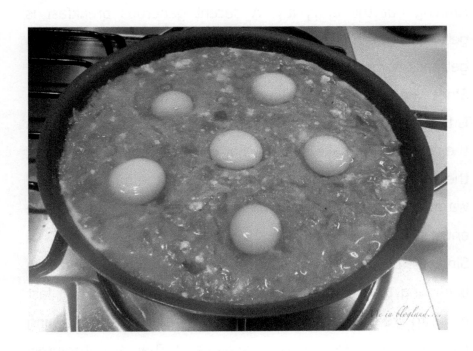

DENVER EGG MUFFINS WITH HAM CRUST

We are arriving at that season where we are preparing spring fever and for the mid-year break. School is drawing nearer to being out and kids are rising later and later for school and running out the entryway. A decent generous breakfast is getting increasingly hard to get a hold of nowadays. My children get back home starving from school.

Since one of our preferred morning meals to make on the blog is this Oven Baked Denver Omelet, I chose to transform it into these simple to make biscuits that can keep going throughout the entire week. You simply pop them into the microwave and warm and have a heavenly breakfast prepared to run out the entryway.

Since we have our eggs conveyed to us every week, they were beginning to accumulate in the ice chest. I was at long last ready to fire spending a portion of those eggs and this morning meal was an extraordinary arrangement! They are absolutely adaptable to your families taste however we love the straightforwardness of peppers, onions, and ham. They are stuffed with season and the ooey gooey cheddar inside is delish!

These are without a doubt the ideal make ahead breakfast biscuits for you or your kiddos in a hurry! Stuffed with protein these healthy Denver omelet breakfast biscuits will turn into a family top pick!

Denver Omelet Breakfast Muffins are such an incredible breakfast and ideal for making ahead or in a hurry! Stacked with Peppers, onions, ham and ooey gooey cheddar, these will turn into a top pick!

Fixings

½ cup onion hacked

1 cup green pepper hacked

1 cup hacked completely cooked ham

1 cup destroyed cheddar

8 eggs

½ cup creamer cream

1 teaspoon salt

1/4 teaspoon pepper

Cut green onion for trimming (or you can include it in.)

Directions

Preheat stove to 400 degrees. Gently oil a 12 biscuit skillet. Separation the onion, green pepper, and ham equitably over the 12 biscuit tins. Include the cheddar equitably the top.

In a medium estimated bowl whisk the eggs, creamer, salt and pepper. Pour over the highest point of the cheddar and fill the liner until practically full.

Prepare for 20-22 minutes or until set. Evacuate and serve warm or let cool and store in the fridge or cooler. Warm from refrigerator for around 30 seconds or solidified for around 1 moment or until warmed through.

CHEESY SLOW COOKER EGG CASSEROLE

In some emphasis of my most out of this world fantasies, I walk first floor each morning to locate a beautiful, filling, and healthy breakfast arranged and sitting tight for me. The plates are white, the napkins adorable and vivid, and a stylish bud jar loaded up with new blossoms is at the focal point of the table. While I won't be experienced my tablescape dreams at any point in the near future, I do have a formula that will make you have a feeling that you have an individual breakfast cook: Crockpot Egg Casserole!

I was going to type "a formula that will make you sense that you've requested room administration" rather, yet since the ideal area for cooking a moderate cooker egg goulash medium-term is likely your kitchen, the similarity didn't exactly apply.

I do lament that you should stroll from your room to the kitchen to appreciate it. I guarantee the slight bother will merit your exertion!

As somebody who gets up each morning prepared to eat at the present time (and who wouldn't believe herself to pursue a formula until espresso has reestablished her to a fundamental degree of usefulness), I relish make-ahead simple slow cooker breakfast meal plans like this one.

During the week, I keep it straightforward with medium-term steel cut oats (for a hot form, see these medium-term moderate cooker steel cut oats). Ends of the week, in any case, leave me wanting something heartier and increasingly liberal.

What about making a medium-term slow cooker breakfast with bacon, gooey fontina cheddar, and vegetables for shading + justification of additional servings? I don't think about you, however that is my concept of a Saturday or Sunday morning lived without limit.

Why I Love This Easy Egg Casserole

Ben and I don't go out for breakfast or early lunch often, to a limited extent because I ordinarily appreciate the morning meals we cook at home more.

Making your own early lunch is a simple method to set aside cash, and since breakfast plans are commonly too basic, you needn't bother with a lot of understanding to pull off something café commendable in any case.

I additionally love to dodge long end of the week informal breakfast hold up times, which I see as the most difficult of all café pauses. Nobody has eaten at this point day, so when we're situated, have discussed the menu and put in a request, and the nourishment has shown up, a couple of us (ahem, me) will in general be genuinely feisty.

You won't need to look out for this simple simmering pot breakfast meal. The prep occurs in the prior night, so toward the beginning of the day, it's prepared the minute you are!

What is a Crockpot Casserole?

A simmering pot meal is much the same as some other goulash you would make in the stove, yet it's cooked low and slow in the stewing pot. It additionally requires less involved tending than heated meal plans.

For a morning meal slow cooker dish, you can prepare everything the prior night, and a healthy simmering pot breakfast will be sitting tight for you when you wake up.

How would You Know When an Egg Casserole is Done?

When your egg dish is done, it ought to be obviously brilliant around the edges, and the eggs should look firm and set.

The most idiot proof strategy for knowing if an egg goulash is done is by checking the inner temperature with a moment read thermometer or by embeddings a knife in the inside and checking whether it tells the truth.

What temperature should an egg goulash be cooked to? An egg dish ought to be cooked to 160 degrees F.

Making the Best Overnight Crockpot Breakfast Egg Casserole

This medium-term breakfast formula is a super-stacked, flavorful variant of a simmering pot breakfast French toast. Like medium-term French toast dishes (this medium-term blueberry French toast being an undisputed top choice), it utilizes 3D squares of bread and is topped with a blend of eggs and milk.

Rather than sweet or fruity fixings, be that as it may, this stewing pot egg dish is exquisite. It utilizes fixings that you'd find in an exemplary egg prepare, frittata, or omelet.

The Ingredients

Eggs. What would you be able to do with heaps of eggs? All things considered, this formula utilizes 12 (!!) enormous eggs, so making slow cooker egg dish is absolutely my first decision.

Cheddar. Utilize one "melty" cheddar and one "brittle" cheddar for a decent variety of surfaces and flavors. I selected fontina for the melty cheddar and feta for the brittle. For the melty cheddar, cheddar, Swiss, or mozzarella would be incredible decisions. For the brittle, I presume goat cheddar would be stunning.

Vegetables. I gave the formula a Mediterranean turn with artichokes (the canned kind are ultra helpful and immaculate here), spinach (solidified hacked spinach keeps it speedy and simple), and a sweet red chime pepper.

Bacon. Ensured to make any day feel like the end of the week. While egg meal with bacon is my top choice, you can swap disintegrated frankfurter or cubed ham if you like.

Bread. A roll or craftsman sourdough portion is my top pick. If you utilize an entire grain alternative, ensure the flavor of the wheat isn't excessively articulated or it will surpass the more fragile kinds of the vegetables and cheeses.

Many breakfast dishes swap solidified potatoes for the bread. By and by, I love the fleecy, custardy, wanton surface you get with bread and bread alone, so I took the simmering pot egg dish no hash tans approach.

Dijon Mustard + Cayenne. A tad bit of every include profundity and gives the egg dish a genuine "I could be eating this in an eatery" impact.

The Directions

Line your moderate cooker with a dispensable liner. You'll be happy you did this.

Sauté the bacon on the stove, then evacuate to a paper-towel-lined plate. Keep 1 tablespoon drippings in the skillet.

Add the pepper and shallot to the container, and cook until softened.

In a major bowl, whisk the eggs, milk, mustard, and flavors until consolidated.

Layer the bread, sautéed vegetables, and melty cheddar in the moderate cooker. Top with much more cheddar.

Gradually pour the egg blend over the entirety of the fixings, and sprinkle the bacon on top.

Cook for 7 to 8 hours on LOW. Evacuate the goulash to a plate (still in the liner). Let cool, then evacuate the liner. Cut and serve. Appreciate!

Making the Best Overnight Crockpot Breakfast Egg Casserole

This medium-term breakfast formula is a super-stacked, appetizing rendition of a stewing pot breakfast French toast. Like medium-term French toast meals (this medium-term blueberry French toast being an undisputed top choice), it utilizes 3D squares of bread and is topped with a blend of eggs and milk.

Rather than sweet or fruity fixings, in any case, this simmering pot egg meal is flavorful. It utilizes fixings that you'd find in an exemplary egg heat, frittata, or omelet.

The Ingredients

Eggs. What would you be able to do with bunches of eggs? All things considered, this formula utilizes 12 (!!) huge eggs, so making stewing pot egg meal is unquestionably my first decision.

Cheddar. Utilize one "melty" cheddar and one "brittle" cheddar for a decent variety of surfaces and flavors. I settled on fontina for the melty cheddar and feta for the brittle. For the melty cheddar, cheddar, Swiss, or mozzarella would be brilliant decisions. For the brittle, I speculate goat cheddar would be choice.

Vegetables. I gave the formula a Mediterranean curve with artichokes (the canned kind are ultra helpful and impeccable here), spinach (solidified cleaved spinach keeps it brisk and simple), and a sweet red ringer pepper.

Bacon. Ensured to make any day feel like the end of the week. While egg goulash with bacon is my top pick, you can swap disintegrated frankfurter or cubed ham if you like.

Bread. A roll or craftsman sourdough portion is my top choice. If you utilize an entire grain alternative, ensure the flavor of the wheat isn't excessively articulated or it will surpass the more fragile kinds of the vegetables and cheeses.

Many breakfast goulashes swap solidified potatoes for the bread. By and by, I love the cushy, custardy, wanton surface you get with bread and bread alone, so I took the slow cooker egg meal no hash tans approach.

Dijon Mustard + Cayenne. A tad bit of every include profundity and gives the egg meal a genuine "I could be eating this in an eatery" impact.

The Directions

Line your moderate cooker with an expendable liner. You'll be happy you did this.

Sauté the bacon on the stove, then expel to a paper-towel-lined plate. Keep 1 tablespoon drippings in the skillet.

Add the pepper and shallot to the dish, and cook until softened. In a major bowl, whisk the eggs, milk, mustard, and flavors until fused.

Layer the bread, sautéed vegetables, and melty cheddar in the moderate cooker. Top with considerably more cheddar.

Gradually pour the egg blend over the entirety of the fixings, and sprinkle the bacon on top.

Cook for 7 to 8 hours on LOW. Expel the meal to a plate (still in the liner). Let cool, then expel the liner. Cut and serve. Appreciate!

How would You Store Egg Casserole?

To Store. Store egg goulash in a sealed shut stockpiling compartment in the cooler for as long as 3 days.

To Reheat. Warm goulash in a meal or comparable heating dish in the broiler at 350 degrees F until hot. You can likewise tenderly rewarm remains in the microwave on a microwave-safe plate until warmed through.

To Freeze. You can solidify an egg dish! Spot remaining meal in a sealed shut cooler safe stockpiling compartment in the cooler for as long as 2 months. You can likewise wrap singular segments and stop them so you can defrost each segment in turn. Let defrost medium-term in the cooler before warming.

To Make Ahead. If the goulash completes before you are prepared to serve it, you can rewarm singular servings in the microwave or spot the entire thing in a heating dish, spread it with foil, and warm it in the broiler.

What Can You Bring to a Breakfast Potluck?

While this stewing pot egg dish is impeccable to bring to a potluck without anyone else's input, here are a couple of proposals of what else you could carry with it:

Bacon. For a definitive meat-darlings breakfast, serve some Baked Bacon with this goulash.

Potatoes. Egg meal with potatoes would be heavenly. These Crockpot Breakfast Potatoes are constantly a hit at a potluck. You could likewise serve egg goulash with hash tans as an afterthought.

Scones. Serve your stewing pot breakfast dish with bread rolls (like these Easy Drop Biscuits) for a scrumptious, extra-filling spread.

Suggested Tools for Making Slow Cooker Egg Casserole

Slow Cooker. This adaptation changes to "keep warm" to dissuade overcooking.

Slow Cooker Liner. Helps prevent the meal from adhering to your moderate cooker.

Moment Read Thermometer. The most ideal approach to tell if your goulash is finished.

(Nearly) room administration, at your administration!

MAKE-AHEAD BREAKFAST BURRITOS

Fixings

1 pound mass pork hotdog

1-1/2 cups solidified cubed hash dark colored potatoes

1/4 cup diced onion

1/4 cup diced green or red pepper

4 huge eggs, gently beaten

12 flour tortillas (8 inches), warmed

1/2 cup Kerrygold destroyed cheddar

Picante sauce and sharp cream, discretionary

Bearings

In a huge skillet, cook wiener over medium warmth until never again pink; channel. Include the potatoes, onion and pepper; cook and mix for 6-8 minutes or until delicate. Include eggs; cook and mix until set.

Spoon filling askew on every tortilla. Sprinkle with cheddar. Overlay sides and finishes over topping and move off. Present with picante sauce and harsh cream if wanted.

To solidify and warm burritos: Wrap every burrito in waxed paper and foil. Stop for as long as multi month. To utilize, expel foil and waxed paper. Spot one burrito on a microwave-safe plate. Microwave on high for 2 to 2-1/4 minutes or until a thermometer peruses 165°, turning burrito over once. Let represent 20 seconds.

BREAKFAST PIZZA

If cold extra pizza is a morning meal you'd preferably leave as a school memory, however the possibility of pizza for breakfast still interests, then this formula is for you. You can discover breakfast pizza practically anyplace, however there's a variant well known in the Midwest that we're entirely stricken with. This local strength may appear to be standard from the outset — frankfurter, eggs, and cheddar on a fundamental outside — yet when you look nearer, you'll locate a smooth cheddar sauce instead of a random bunch of cheddar, and hash tans took care of under the layer of meat and eggs. It's those subtleties that make this corner store pizza one to be motivated by.

While you can make the whole pizza from beginning to end in about an hour on an end of the week morning, you can likewise make the vast majority of the fixings the prior night and heat this pizza up in under 30 minutes anytime.

So how would you make a pizza for breakfast? The appropriate response is the basic one you're expecting: Top it with standard breakfast passage, yet do it with some artfulness. Our own gets frankfurter, hash tans, and fried eggs because it's generous, scrumptious, and warms well. This formula peruses long, yet you can make the cheddar sauce, cook the wiener and eggs, and mesh the cheddar the prior night and simply collect the pizza the following day.

Beating Shortcuts

Cheddar sauce: You can make the cheddar sauce the prior night and store it in an impenetrable holder. Or on the other hand don't hesitate to utilize a readied item, for example, Cheese-Wiz.

Wiener: Bulk breakfast frankfurter is the best approach here. Concoct it the prior night.

Eggs: I'm typically not a backer for cooking fried eggs ahead of time, yet between the cheddar sauce and the cheddar on top, the pre-cooked eggs will steam to warm and won't dry out in the stove. These can be cooked the prior night also.

Solidified hash tans: While custom made hash tans are more delectable, utilizing solidified hash darker potatoes and defrosting them in the refrigerator medium-term will spare significant planning time.

Utilizing Leftovers

Breakfast pizza is an extraordinary method to go through scraps. Solid shape extra frittata (or breakfast dish) and put that on the pizza rather than the fried eggs, or swap the hash tans for remaining cooked vegetables from the previous evening's supper. The equation of pizza covering + cheddar sauce + cheddar + fixings will make those remains energizing once more.

Step by step instructions to Make Breakfast Pizza

SERVES

6 to 8

Fixings

Cooking shower

1 tablespoon unsalted margarine

1 tablespoon universally handy flour

1/4 cups entire milk, isolated

3/4 cup destroyed cheddar, isolated

1/2 teaspoon fit salt, isolated

8 ounces uncooked breakfast frankfurter, housings evacuated

4 enormous eggs

1 pound pizza mixture, at room temperature

1 cup solidified hash darker potatoes, defrosted

1 cup destroyed mozzarella cheddar

2 scallions, meagerly cut

Hardware

Heating sheet

Little pan

Whisk

Blending bowl

Medium nonstick griddle

Paper towel

Guidelines

Warmth the broiler. Mastermind a rack in the broiler and warmth to 375°F. Coat a heating sheet with cooking splash.

Make the cheddar sauce. Soften the margarine in a little pot over medium-high warmth. Include the flour and cook, mixing, until the margarine flour blend loses its sheen, around 1 moment. Rush in 1 cup of the milk and heat to the point of boiling, whisking once in a while, until thickened, 3 to 4 minutes. Expel from the warmth and rush in 1/2 cup of the cheddar and 1/4 teaspoon of the salt. Put aside to cool somewhat while you make the remainder of the fixings.

Cook the wiener and eggs. Warmth a medium nonstick griddle over medium-high warmth. Disintegrate the hotdog into the container and cook until seared and cooked through, 5 to 7 minutes. While the hotdog cooks, whisk together the eggs, staying 1/4 cup of milk, and staying 1/4 teaspoon salt in a medium bowl. Utilize an opened spoon to move the cooked hotdog to a paper towel-lined plate. Leave the hotdog's fat in the dish and pour in the egg blend. Scramble the eggs until nearly cooked through yet at the same time wet, 3 to 4 minutes. Expel the container from the warmth.

Roll and dock the pizza mixture. Roll or stretch the pizza mixture out into a 12-inch round. Move the mixture to the heating sheet. Utilize the tines of a fork to "dock" (jab gaps in) the pizza mixture, working from the center out to inside 1 inch of the edge. This will keep the batter from getting wet from the steaming cheddar sauce.

Sauce the pizza. Spread on the cheddar sauce in a far, even layer as you would pizza sauce. You probably won't utilize all the cheddar sauce.

Top the pizza. Sprinkle the hotdog onto the cheddar sauce, trailed by the hash tans, lastly the fried eggs. Sprinkle the pizza with the mozzarella cheddar, staying 1/4 cup of cheddar, and scallions.

Prepare for 20 to 25 minutes. Heat until the cheddar is softened and the outside layer is brilliant dark colored, 20 to 25 minutes.

Cool and cut. Let the pizza cool for 10 minutes; this gives the cheddar sauce time to set and keep it from overflowing out. Move to a cutting board, cut, and serve.

Formula NOTES

Capacity: Leftover pizza can be put away firmly enclosed by the cooler for as long as 3 days. Warm in a stove or toaster broiler for best outcomes.

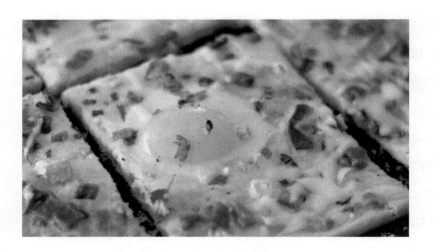

FARMERS' MARKET SCRAMBLE

Fixings

4 enormous eggs

1 bundle green onions

1/4 cup oil-pressed sun-dried tomatoes, slashed

1/3 cup cremini mushrooms, cut

1/4 cup marinated artichoke hearts, cleaved

1/3 cup rich goat cheddar, isolated into little spoonfuls

Salt and pepper to taste

Hot sauce (I favor Louisiana Hot Sauce) to taste

Headings

Get ready vegetables and put in a safe spot.

Whisk together eggs, salt and pepper in a little bowl. Join vegetables and move to a warmed fry skillet. Scramble blend on medium warmth until fried eggs start to shape.

While for the most part mixed yet at the same time somewhat fluid, include goat cheddar spoonfuls and crease until there are little pockets of cheddar all through. Try not to let cheddar soften totally - you need to see the pockets in your scramble.

Expel from heat, include hot sauce if wanted and serve.

RASPBERRY-LEMON GLUTEN-FREE MUFFINS

It's been momentarily since I posted a gluten free formula; I am so sorry my companions! These Gluten Free Lemon Raspberry Muffins are my new most loved gluten free formula. I love biscuits, particularly with my enormous frosted latte I drink day by day. I have such huge numbers of biscuit plans on my blog, I thought it was time that I made a gluten free form for you.

I have a feeling that I have discovered gold. A gluten free biscuit loaded with season, with a decent arch and you may never realize it was without gluten. Notwithstanding testing them myself, I've approached my gluten free companions for input and their outcomes were reliable: the berries are tart, and the biscuits are damp and superior to anything what they have found in the normal pastry kitchen.

I have attempted a couple of different gluten free flours and I need to state my favored image is King Arthur Flour. It's a mixed flour blend that can be fill in for ordinary flour. Notwithstanding, remember to include the thickener, or your biscuits will be extremely runny. Regardless they taste fine, yet they are definitely not as lovely. I can disclose to you that from direct understanding.

This ace biscuit formula can be effectively fill in for an assortment of flavors or organic products. If you don't care for lemon, you can overlook the lemon totally. You can substitute the raspberries for blackberries or blueberries as well! The almond concentrate can likewise be fill in for vanilla or different flavors.

At first I didn't know if the gluten free flour would respond the equivalent in preparing to give me a pleasant round, high vault. By pre-warming your broiler to be exceptionally hot (425°F), and preparing at the high temperature for a couple of moments, it will enable the biscuits to rise. Then following five minutes, you can decrease the warmth to 350°F. Science rises to the ideal arch, and everybody realizes the biscuit tops are the best part!

Fixings

9 oz Fresh raspberries, flushed

2 1/2 C Gluten free flour (King Arthur brand is liked)

1/2 tsp Xanthan gum

1 C Granulated sugar

4 tsp Baking powder

1/2 tsp Salt

1 Large egg

1 C Buttermilk or milk

1/2 C Butter (liquefied)

1/4 C Sour cream

1 tsp Almond remove

1 tbsp Lemon juice (new crushed)

Get-up-and-go from 1 lemon

Directions

Wash and flush raspberries. Use ¼ C of gluten free flour to cover the raspberries. Tenderly mix to cover the raspberries in flour. Put in a safe spot.

Preheat broiler to 425°.

In a medium-sized bowl, measure out 2 ¼ cups of gluten free flour with thickener. Include sugar, preparing powder and salt. Mix to consolidate and afterward put this blend in a safe spot.

In a medium-sized bowl, beat the egg utilizing a race until light and feathery. Gather buttermilk and dissolved margarine and rush into a single unit with the egg. Then include almond concentrate, and sharp cream and whisk everything together until smooth.

Include new crushed lemon squeeze and get-up-and-go into wet blend and rush until joined.

Gradually empty wet fixings into the dry fixings and utilize a wooden spoon to blend just until joined. Your hitter will be thicker, yet cautious not to over blend! In conclusion, overlap in the raspberries. Try not to pour in the abundance flour extra from the berries.

Line your biscuit skillet and fill your biscuit liners right to the top with hitter. Sprinkle with cut almonds.

Prepare for 5 minutes at 425° and afterward lessen warmth to 350° and heat for another 16-20 minutes. Try not to open the broiler for at any rate 15 minutes; you will perceive how pleasantly the biscuits rise. Preparing times will shift by stove.

Check your biscuits for doneness by embeddings a toothpick into the focal point of the biscuit. If your toothpick tells the truth, your biscuit is finished. Enable biscuits to cool totally in the skillet. You can likewise cool on a wire rack, however you need to enable them to sufficiently cool to evacuate and ship them out of the container.

What Can I Substitute in this Gluten Free Easy Lemon Raspberry Muffins Recipe?

Gluten free oat flour: swap with gluten free generally useful flour or natively constructed oat flour.

Whitened almond flour: swap with almond feast, cashew flour or sunflower seed supper.

Non-dairy milk: swap with your preferred veggie lover milk refreshment.

Lemon juice: swap with squeezed orange.

Lemon pizzazz: swap with orange get-up-and-go.

Coconut oil: swap with liquefied veggie lover margarine or flavorless oil.

Coconut sugar: sub with natural dark colored sugar or natural genuine sweetener.

Maple syrup: sub with fluid sugar. Attempt date syrup, agave or nectar (if not veggie lover).

Raspberries: swap with your preferred crisp organic product, similar to blueberries or blackberries, dislike, an entire orange. Hehe!

Note: remember that this formula is made similarly as composed. So any progressions made (little or large) can have a tremendous effect—it's hazardous, people! So try and have a great time, however keep ya head up if it's not great. Simply attempt again or approach me for counsel.

Upbeat Lemon Raspberry Muffins! <—Is it just me or does heating healthy gluten free biscuits simply light up your day? Something about hand crafted can't be beat. Especially when we're preparing with our friends and family. Sending all of you my appreciation for preparing with me. I can hardly wait to hear what you think.

PUMPKINS SPICE MUFFINS

One of the most well-known posts on the blog is our pumpkin bread. In the event that you've made it you know why. Straightforward. Loaded down with pumpkin. Delicate and delicate surface. The best. Clearly we're into breads of late at our home (OK, we're generally into custom made bread). Today I'm sharing a wind on that most loved pumpkin bread formula.

Simple Pumpkin Muffins

These biscuits have a player that will take under 10 minutes to stir up. It's a similar hitter in the pumpkin bread. No progressions to the hitter itself. It needn't bother with any progressions since that bread turns out flawless every.time. What's more, it has exactly the intended effect heated in biscuit tins, as well. Simply take a gander at the tall ascent on these pumpkin biscuits. A perfect domed top

At the point when we initially took a gander at the completed biscuits, Maddie and I stated, "They look simply like Panera's pumpkin biscuits!" I didn't in any capacity expect to make a copycat formula, however in our eyes, these are superior to Panera's pumpkin biscuits.

What's more, here's the reason.

Pumpkin Muffins with Streusel

They're heated with a basic streusel on top. As I would like to think, streusel makes everything better. This specific streusel is made of flour, margarine and sugar. 3 basic fixings that taste so beautiful when prepared into biscuits.

Also, is the powdered sugar vital? I state yes. Not exclusively does the white powdered sugar light up them up, however that smidgen of sweet upgrades the appetizing pumpkin flavors in the biscuit.

Pumpkin Chocolate Chip Muffins

In the event that you love chocolate, take a stab at adding 1 to 1/2 cups smaller than expected chocolate chips to this pumpkin biscuit formula. Overlay in the chocolate chips as the absolute last advance to stirring up the player. Be mindful so as not to over blend! You'll have chocolate in each nibble. Phenomenal!

A pretty introduction and a phenomenal taste!

Pumpkin Spice Muffins

These pumpkin zest biscuits are gently spiced, delicate and sodden. The streusel and powdered sugar on top adds a trace of sweetness to each nibble.

Course Breakfast

Food American

Watchword simple biscuits, pumpkin biscuits, pumpkin zest

Planning Time 15 minutes

Cook Time 15 minutes

All out Time 30 minutes

Servings 18

Calories 253kcal

Creator Julie Clark

Fixings

1 cup canola oil

2 cups granulated sugar

2 teaspoons vanilla

3 enormous eggs

2 cups strong pack pumpkin

3 cups universally handy flour

1 teaspoon salt

1 teaspoon heating pop

2 teaspoons heating powder

2 teaspoons cinnamon

1 teaspoon pumpkin pie zest

Streusel Topping:

3 tablespoons cold margarine

1/2 cup granulated sugar

1/2 cup generally useful flour

1/4 cup powdered sugar

US Customary - Metric

Directions

Preheat the stove to 375 degrees.

Combine the oil, sugar, eggs, vanilla and pumpkin in a bowl. Put in a safe spot. In a different bowl, combine the flour, salt, preparing pop, heating powder, cinnamon and pumpkin pie zest. Add the wet fixings to the dry fixings and blend just until consolidated.

Spoon the player into biscuit dish that have been splashed with cooking shower. Gap the hitter to make 18 biscuits.

In a little bowl, cut the spread into the flour and sugar with a blade and additionally fork. Blend until it looks like scraps and the margarine is in little pieces.

Gap the streusel between the 18 biscuits, sprinkling it over the unbaked mixture.

Prepare the biscuits for 13-15 minutes, until the cupcakes have risen and a toothpick embedded in the inside tells the truth.

Enable the biscuits to cool in the search for gold minutes, at that point evacuate them to a wire rack to cool totally.

When the biscuits are cool, utilize a filtering spoon to filter powdered sugar over top.

The calories indicated depend on the formula making 18 biscuits, with 1 serving being 1 biscuit. Since various brands of fixings have distinctive nourishing data, the calories demonstrated are only a gauge.

You realize what makes an extraordinary fall breakfast, other than pumpkin bread? Pumpkin biscuits. You know what's a far superior breakfast? Streusel-beat pumpkin. In spite of the fact that you might not have given it a shot biscuits, you're presumably acquainted with streusel. Espresso cake, apple fresh (or pumpkin fresh), and disintegrate bested pies are altogether covered with the delicate yet-crunchy blend of spread, flour, and sugar. Here, we've included pumpkin pie flavor also to energize the fall vibes of this morning meal treat. These simple biscuits are likewise really agreeable with regards to changing fixings. No harsh cream? Attempt Greek yogurt or creme fraiche. Not into pumpkin pie flavor? Utilize an equivalent sum (or a mix) of cinnamon, nutmeg, and allspice. Attempt a touch of ground cardamom also for a citrusy, home grown note. Obviously, perhaps the best thing about biscuits is the way that you can without much of a stretch make them ahead. After the biscuits have completely cooled, pack them in cooler safe sacks or compartments and pop them in the cooler. They'll keep going for two-three months, no issue. You can defrost in the cooler for a couple of hours, or all the more rapidly in the microwave, at that point heat them up in the broiler.

Lightning Source UK Ltd.
Milton Keynes UK
UKHW021845100621
385314UK00002B/289